To : Makayla

Challenge yourself with reading and
through reading you will learn.
Never forget you are already special
and can do great things.

Tanya Thompson-Badamosi, MD

To my supportive husband, Akeem, and our precious children–Gianna, Jayden, and Gabriel. You all inspire me every day.

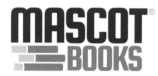

www.mascotbooks.com

Gianna Has Pink Eye

©2018 Dr. Tanya Thompson-Badamosi. All Rights Reserved. No part of this publication may be reproduced, stored in a retrieval system or transmitted in any form by any means electronic, mechanical, or photocopying, recording or otherwise without the permission of the author.

For more information, please contact:
Mascot Books
620 Herndon Parkway, Suite 320
Herndon, VA 20170
info@mascotbooks.com

Library of Congress Control Number: 2018901594

CPSIA Code: PRT0418A
ISBN-13: 978-1-68401-741-6

Printed in the United States

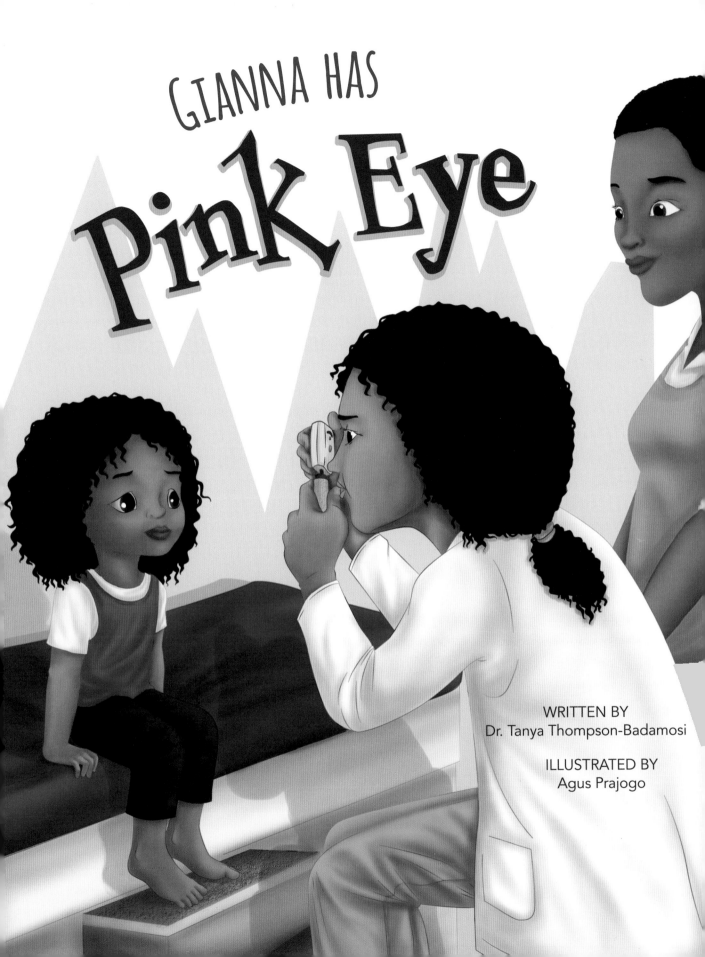

GIANNA HAS
Pink Eye

WRITTEN BY
Dr. Tanya Thompson-Badamosi

ILLUSTRATED BY
Agus Prajogo

Morning came. The sun was up.
It was time to get ready for the day.
"Gianna!" Mom called. "You don't want to be late."
In bed Gianna wanted to stay.

Gianna tossed. Gianna turned.
"Come on, Gianna, open your eyes."
Gianna finally rolled out of bed,
and what a big surprise!

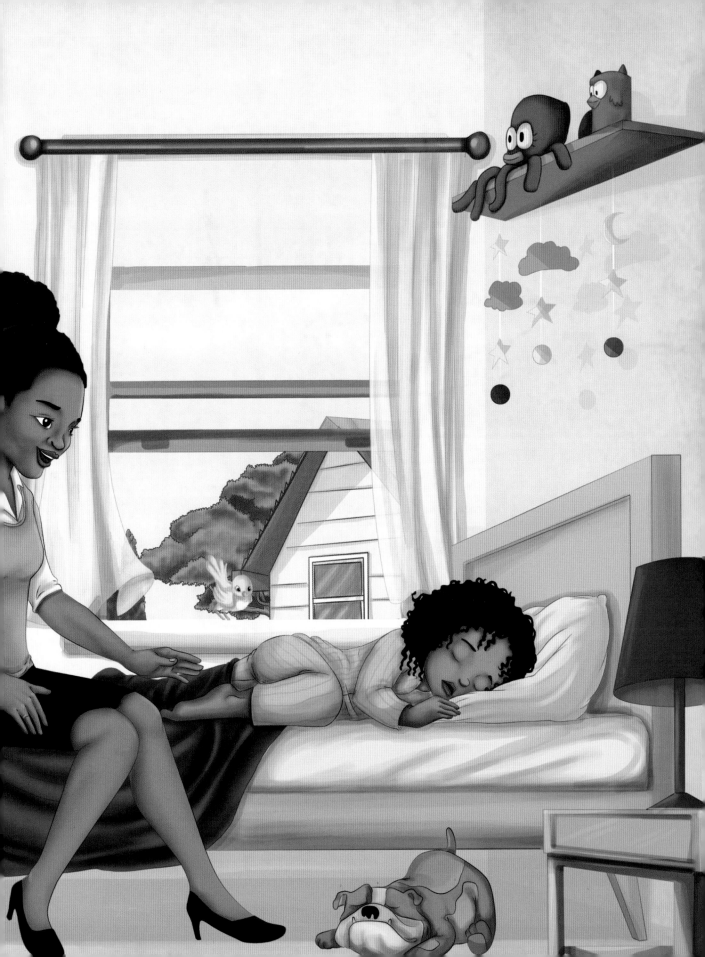

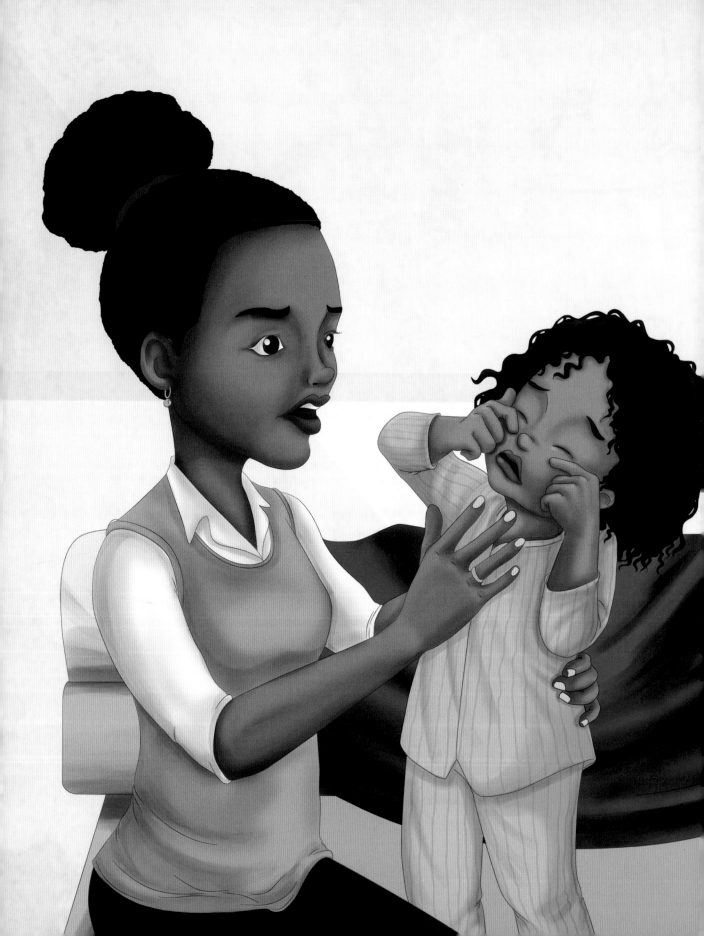

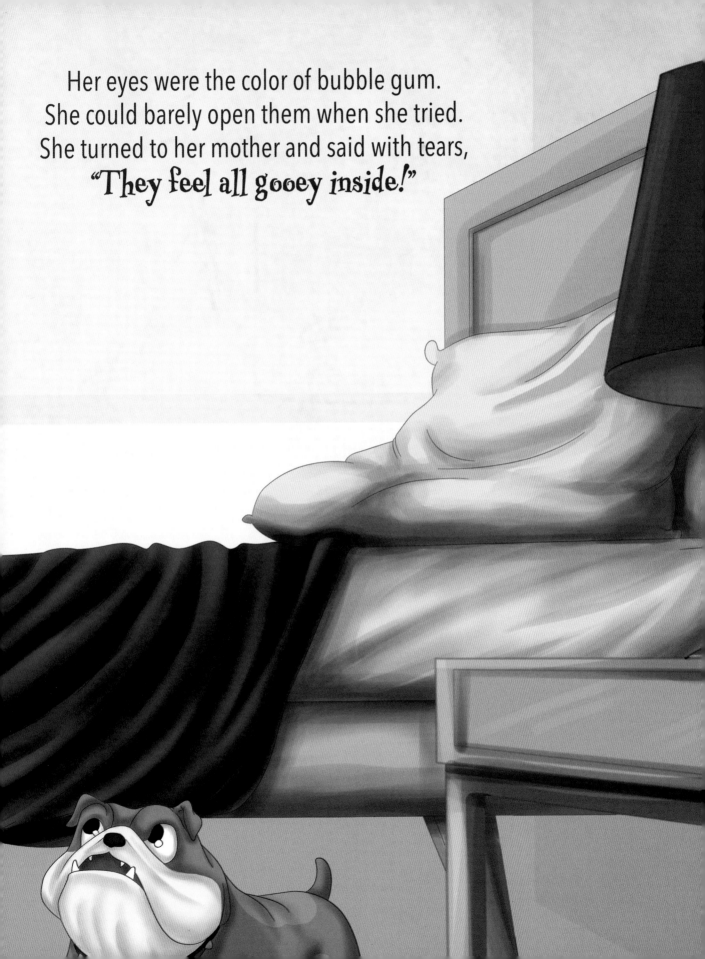

Her eyes were the color of bubble gum.
She could barely open them when she tried.
She turned to her mother and said with tears,
"They feel all gooey inside!"

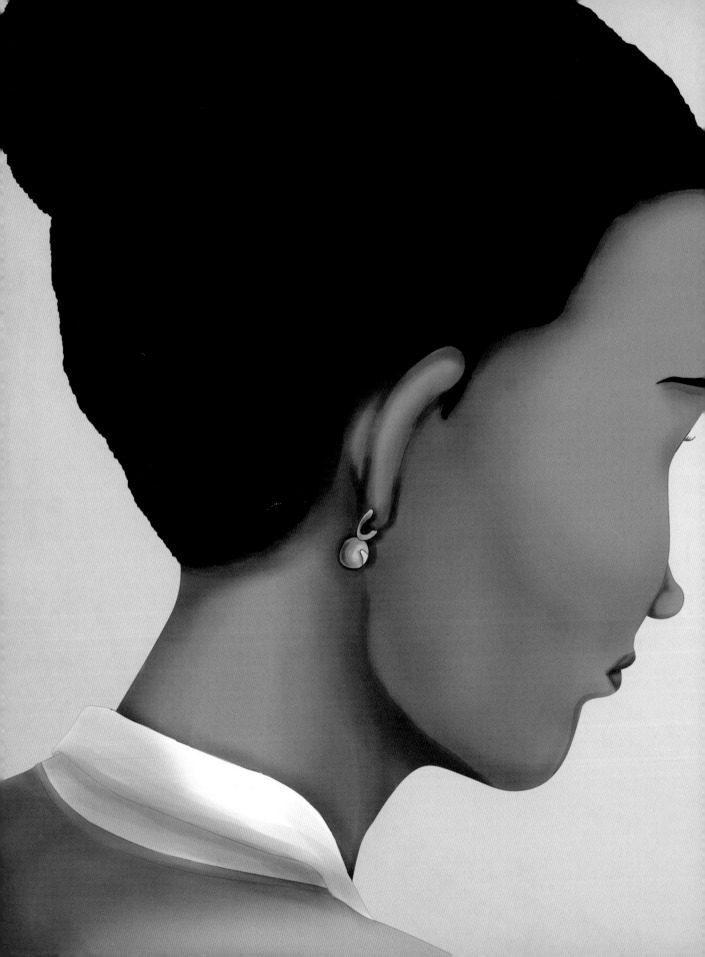

"Oh, wow! Your eyes are pink!
Home you will have to stay.
You have to go to the doctor.
No school for you today."

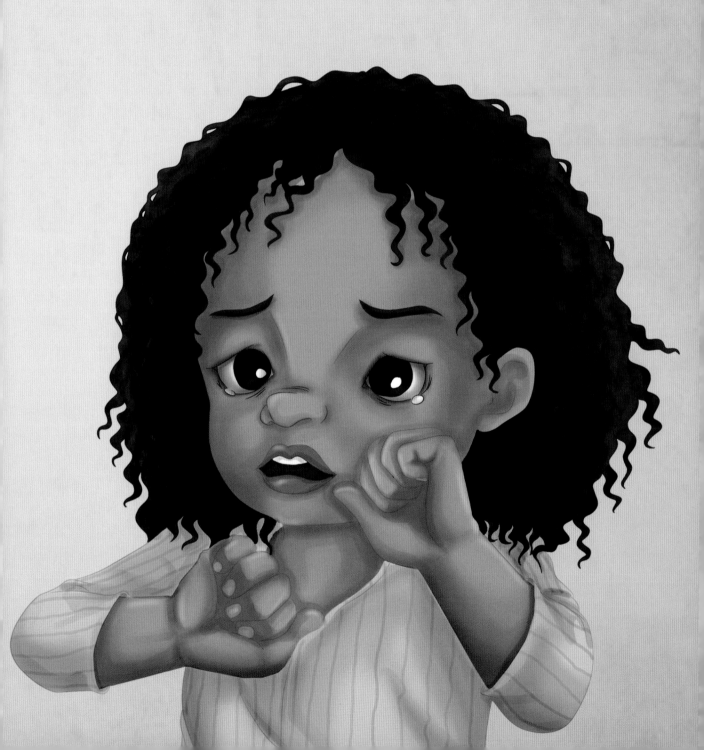

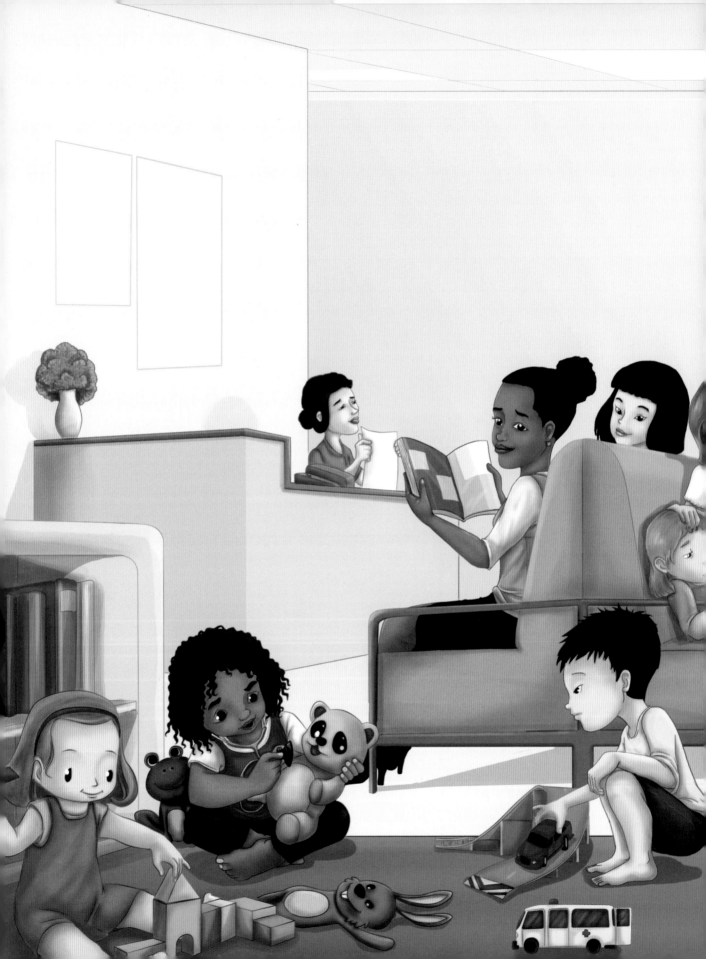

Gianna liked going to the doctor.
She liked looking at her tools.
She liked the doctor listening to her heartbeat.
She makes sure Gianna is healthy for school.

Gianna and her mother waited for Dr. Bee.
They waited to hear Gianna's name called.
The room was filled with books and trains,
cars, a playhouse, and dolls.

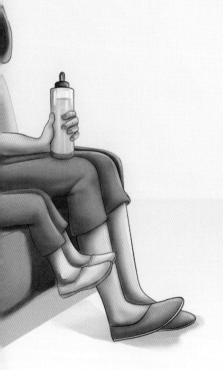
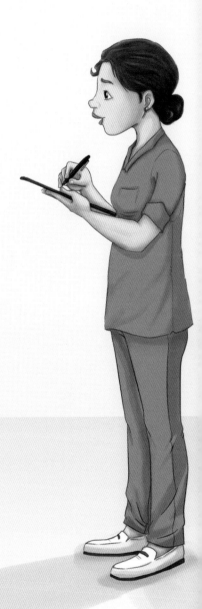

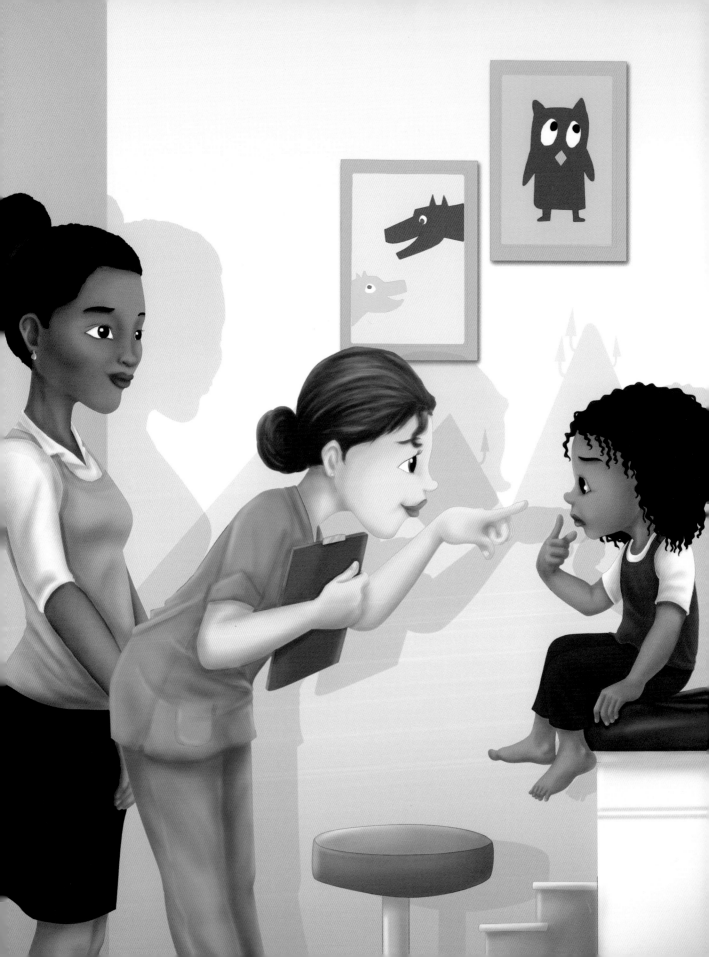

The nurse took Gianna into a room.
"What made you come in today?"
"My eyes are pink and ooey-gooey,
the pink won't go away!"

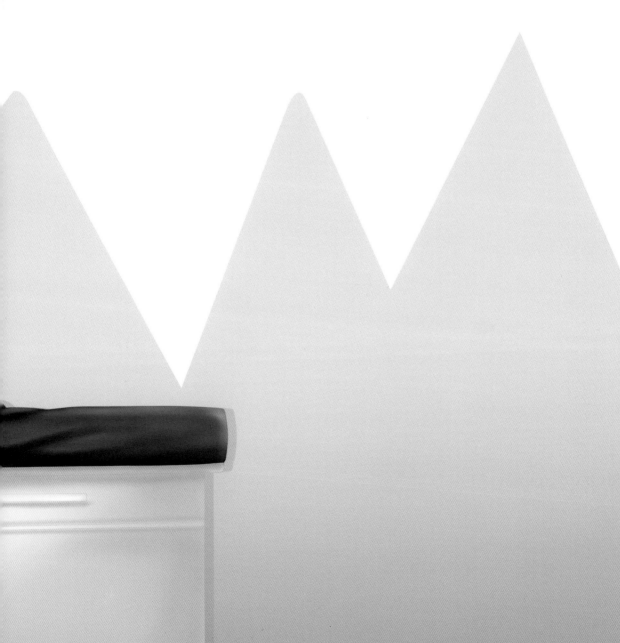

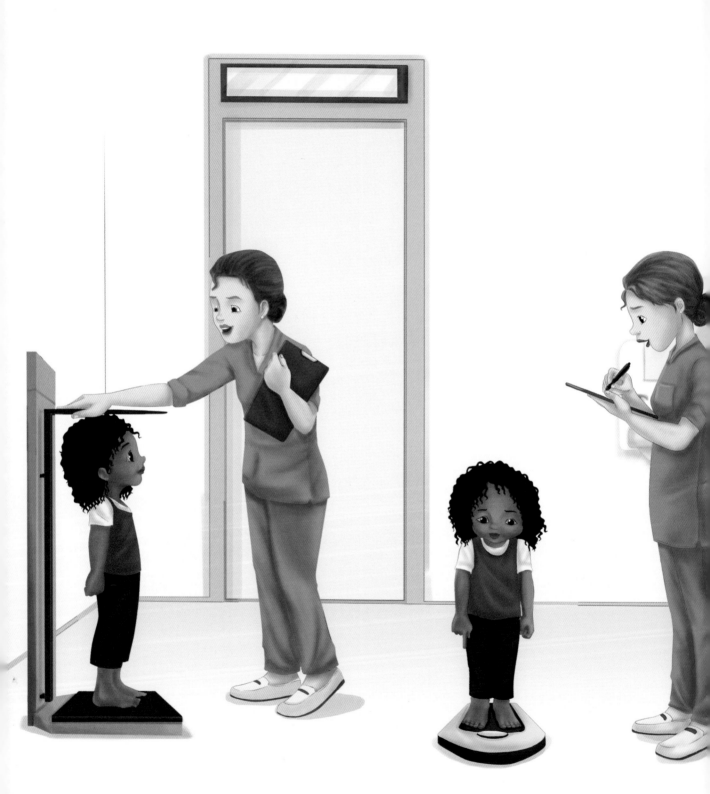

The nurse checked how big Gianna had grown
and put her on a table to sit.
"I'll let the doctor know you're here.
She'll come in a little bit."

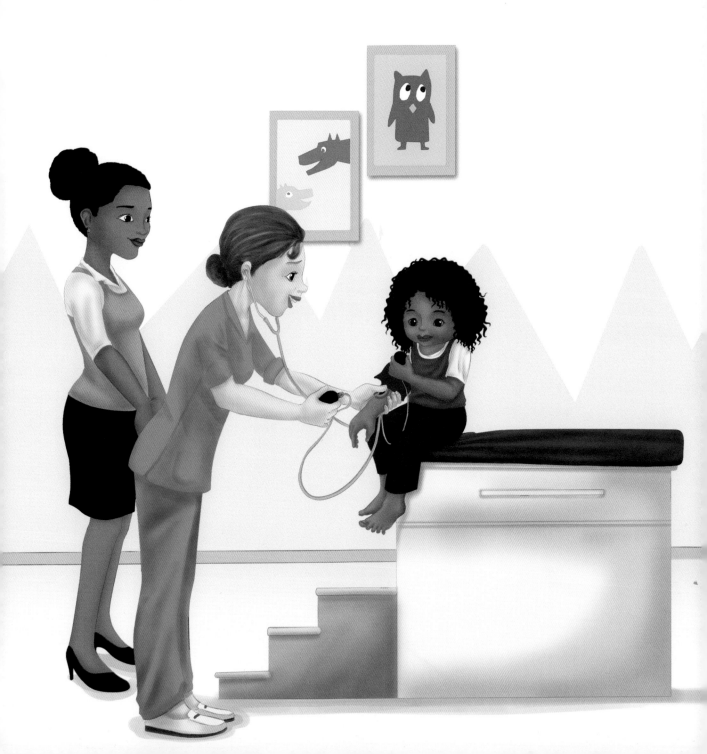

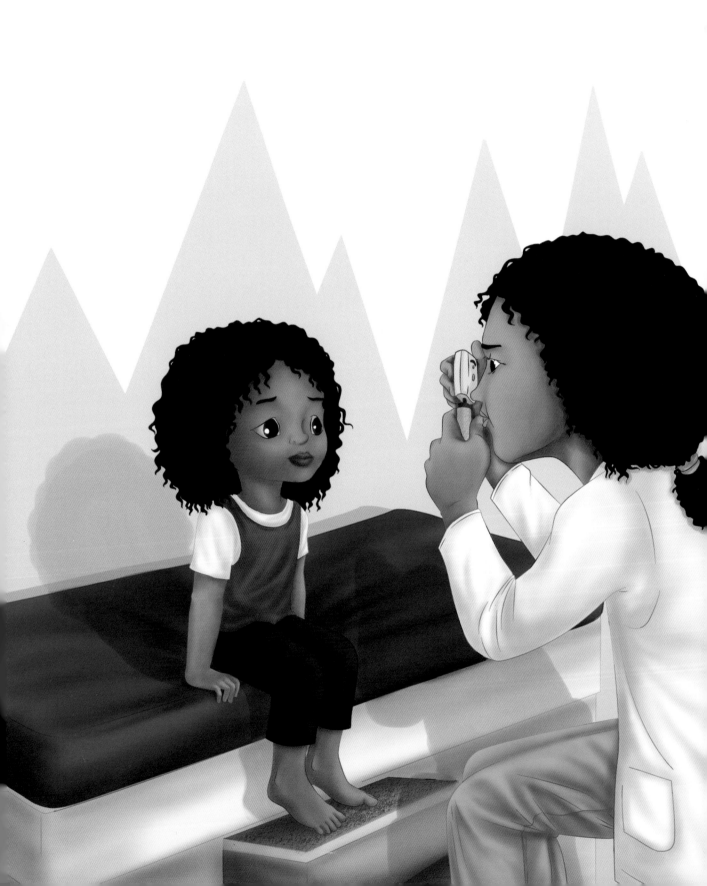

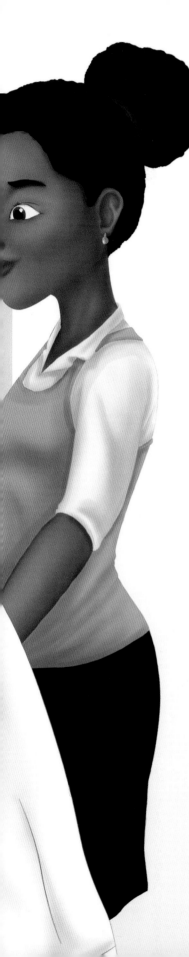

Dr. Bee came into the room.
She smiled and was very nice.
She looked at Gianna's eyes all over,
up, down, left, and right.

"You have pink eye," she said at last.
"It will go away.
You will need to take some medicine,
and stay home from school for the day."

"Wash your hands. Be careful what you touch.
Pink eye spreads fast from one to another.
Everyone in your home can get it—
mother, father, sister, brother!"

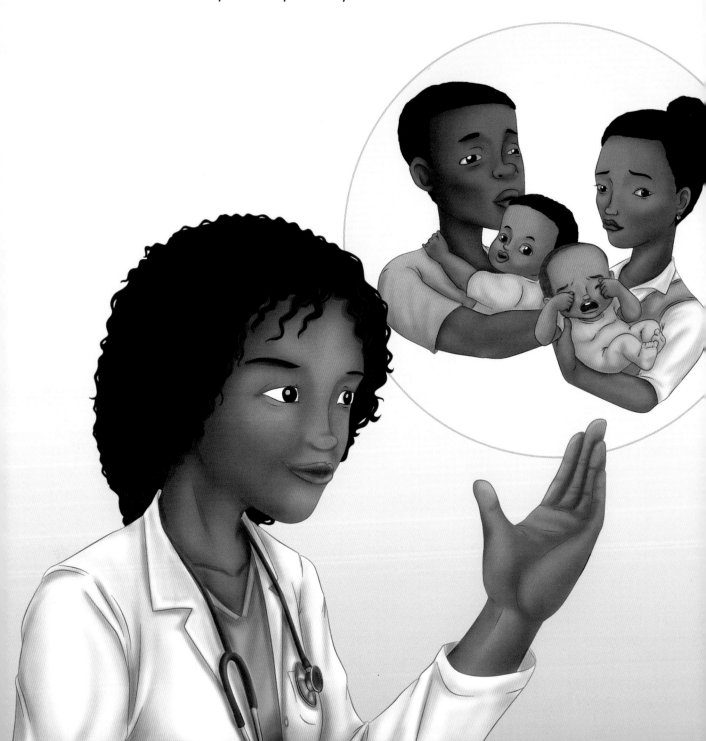

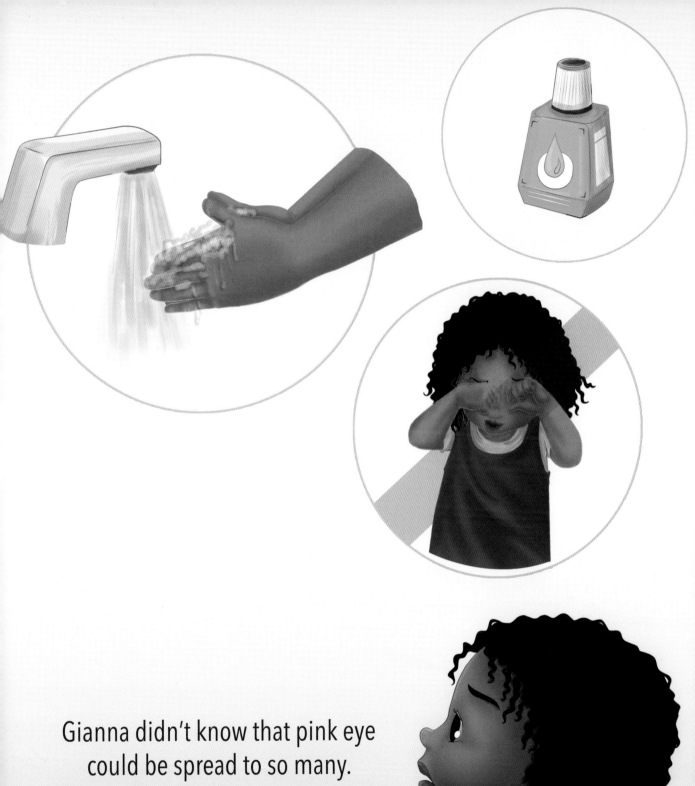

Gianna didn't know that pink eye
could be spread to so many.
She made a vow that, starting now,
she would not spread it any.

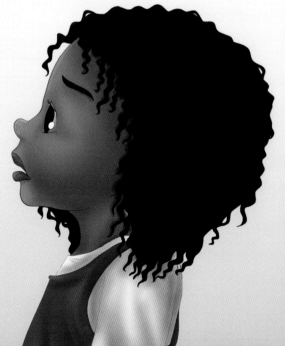

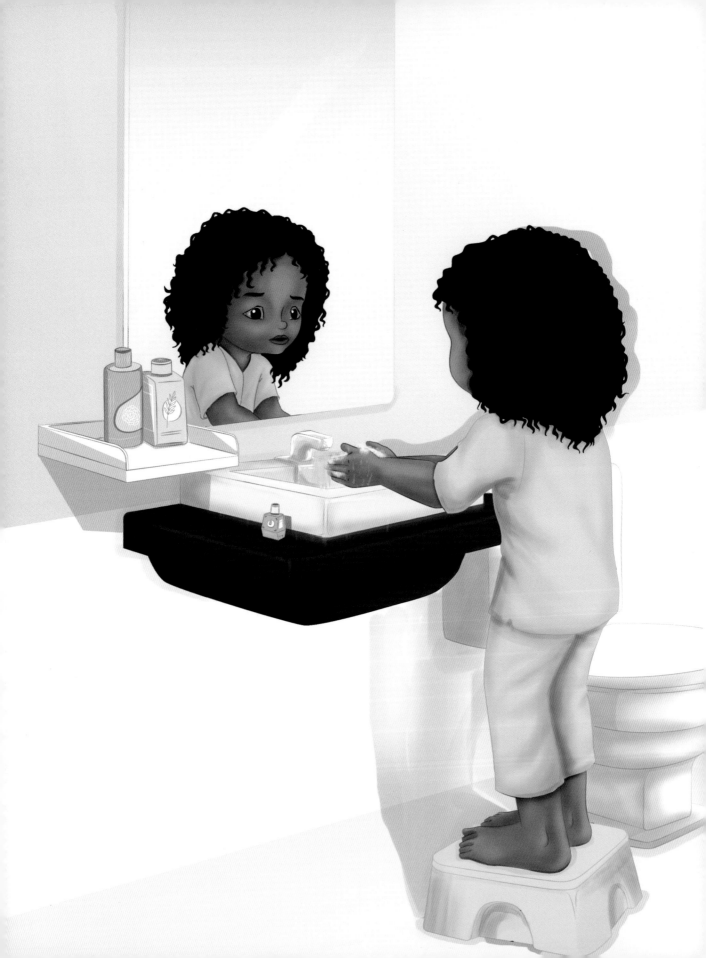

The weekend came and Gianna rested.
She used her eyedrops every day.
She washed her hands and didn't touch her eyes.
She followed Dr. Bee's advice in every way.

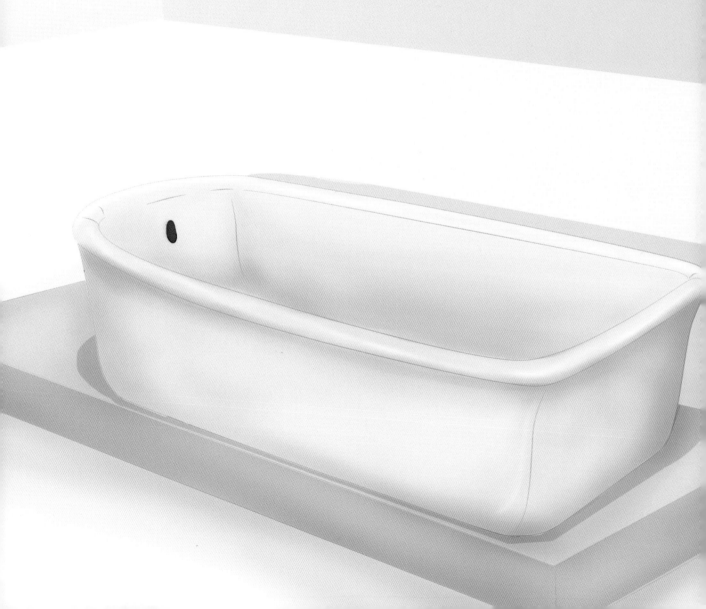

Monday came. The sun was up.
It was time to get ready for the day.
"Gianna!" Mom called. "You don't want to be late."
Gianna shouted, "Hooray!"

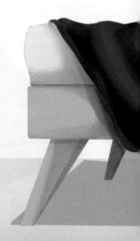

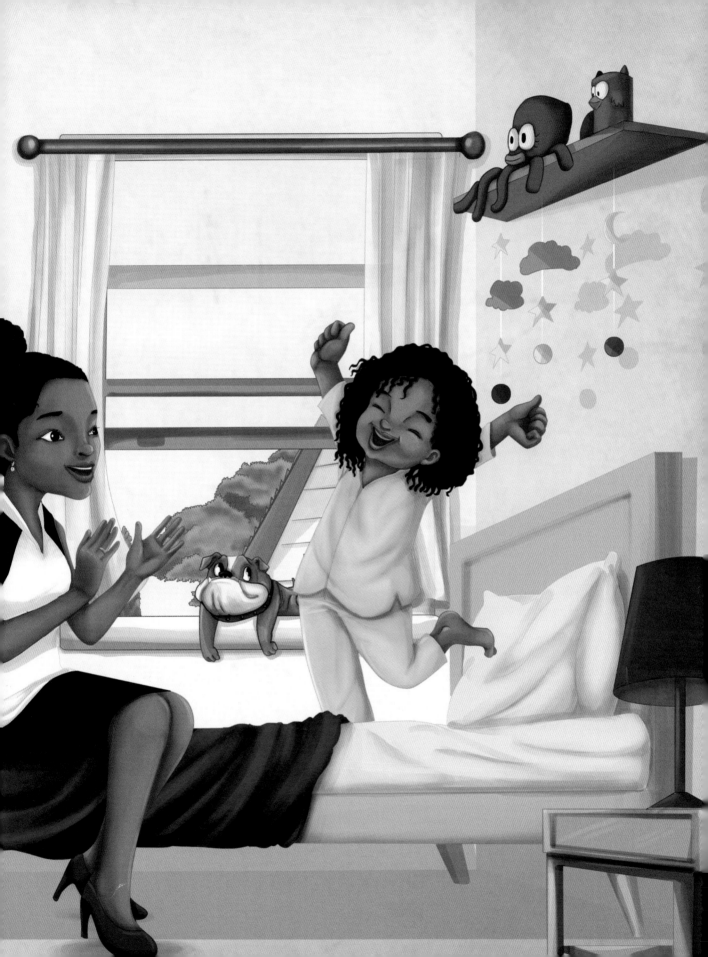

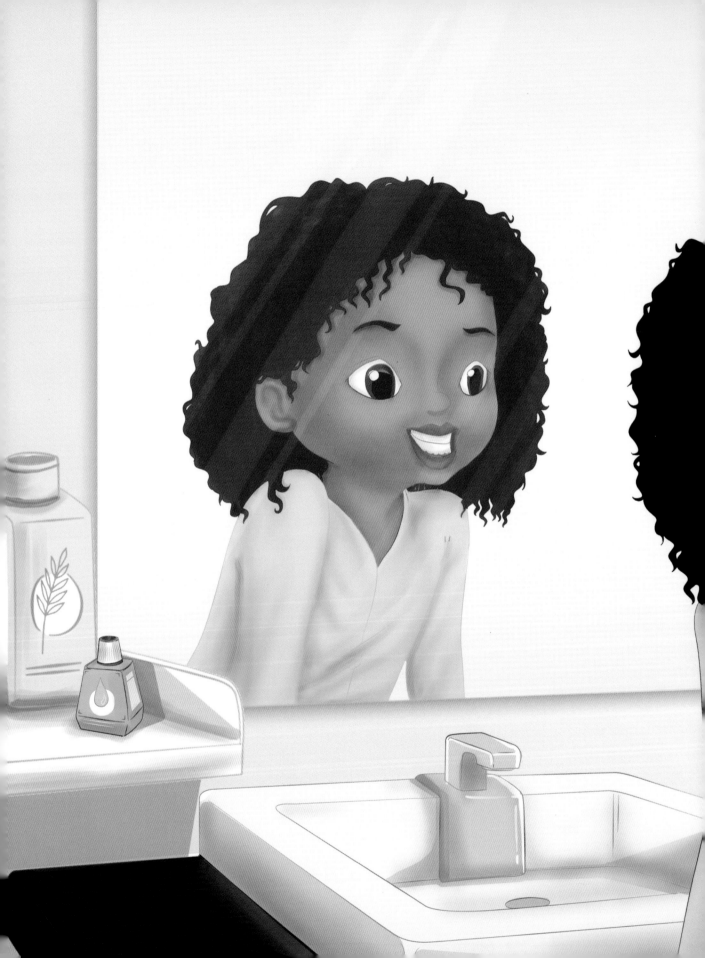

Her eyes were bright! The whites were white.
Gianna could finally see.
Now that her eyes weren't ooey and gooey,
she was as happy as can be.

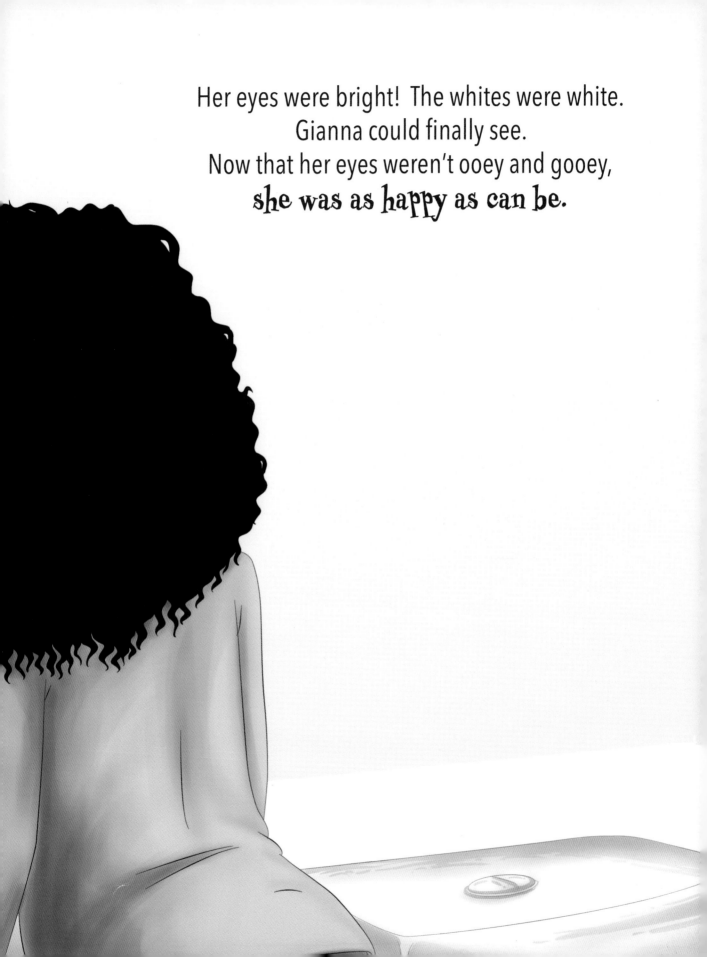

Gianna went to school that day
with no more pink in her eye.
No one else got it either.
She was happy to tell her mom goodbye.

Gianna learned that pink eye comes,
but pink eye does not stay.
And no one else has to get it,
if you protect them in every way.

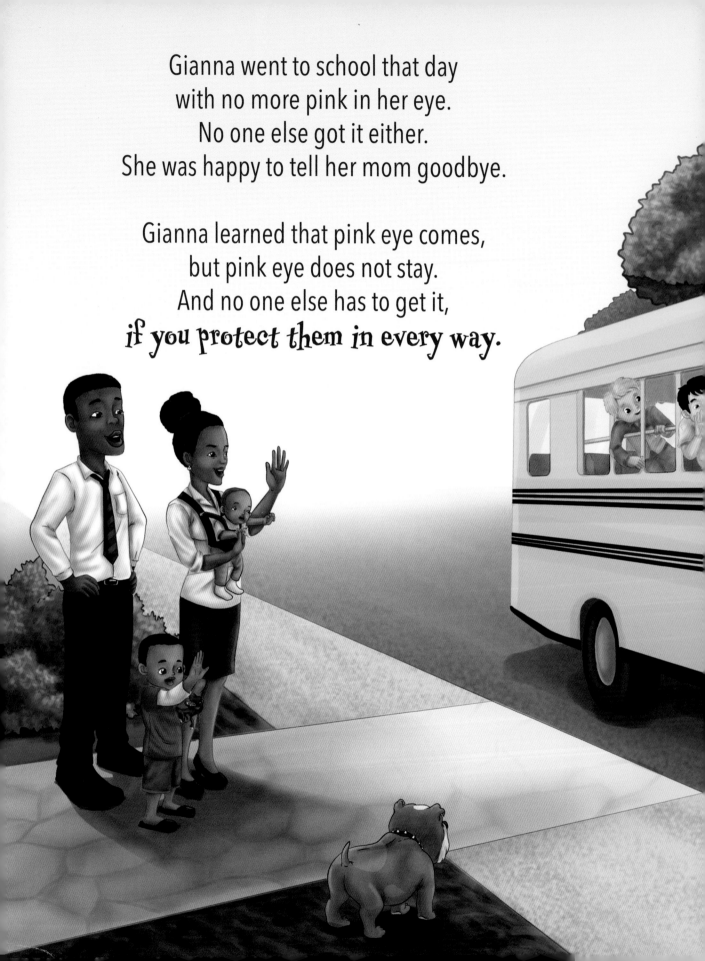

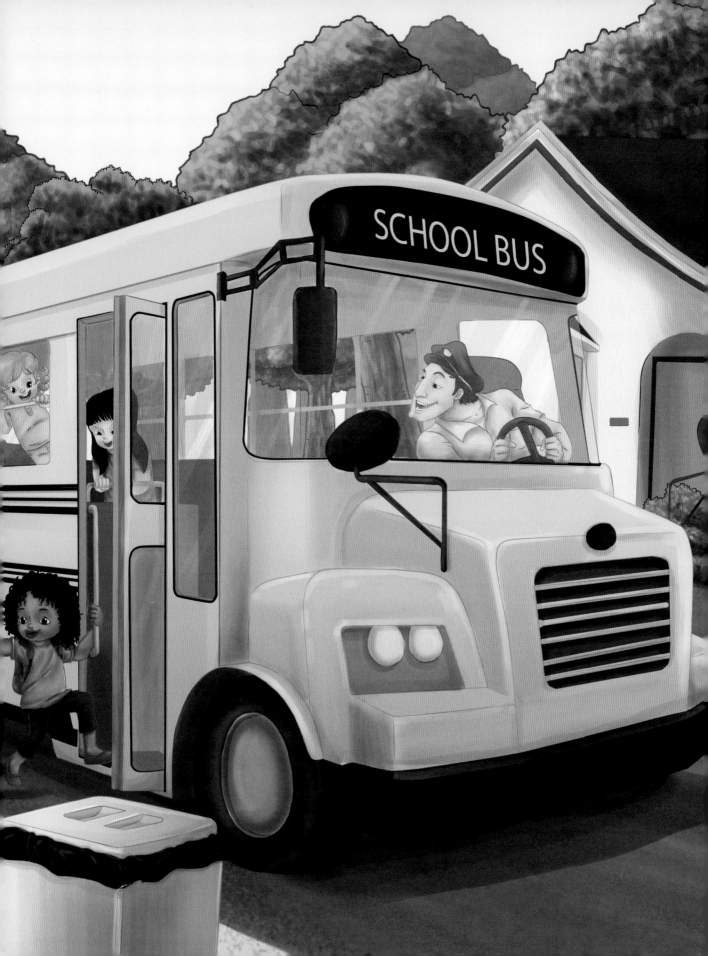

About the Author

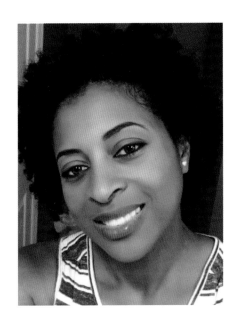

Dr. Tanya Thompson-Badamosi is a physician and fellow of the American College of Endocrinology living in upstate New York. She is the mother of three children and is well-versed in common childhood health concerns. Her oldest child, Gianna, was the inspiration for this book. She enjoys writing, traveling, ice skating, high-intensity interval training, kickboxing, teaching, and relaxing at home (when there is time!). Most of all, she enjoys spending time with her husband and children. Dr. Thompson-Badamosi wrote this book to educate young children about pink eye in an entertaining way. She hopes every young reader and their caregivers will enjoy it!